HOW YOUR BODY WORKS

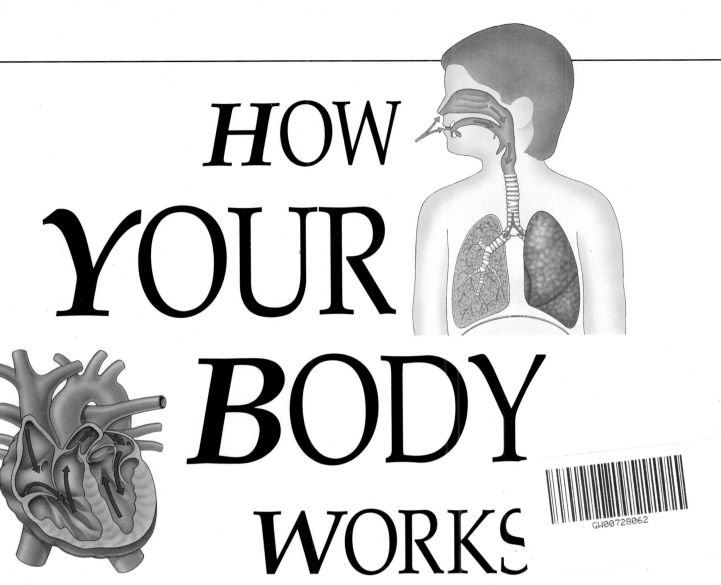

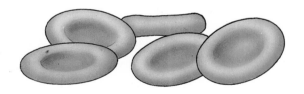

Written by
**Christopher Maynard, Janet De Saulles
and Hazel Songhurst**

Designed by
Chris Leishman

Illustrated by
Kuo Kang Chen
Peter Bull, Jeremy Gower, Christopher Lyon,
Mainline Design

zigzag

About this book

This book was created and produced by Zigzag Publishing Ltd, The Barn, Randolph's Farm, Hurstpierpoint, Sussex BN6 9EL, England

Consultant: Dr Bruce Lambert
Dr Lambert is a GP in a family health centre. He has a special interest in children's health and in health education.

Cover illustrators: Kuo Kang Chen & Peter Bull

Editors: Hazel Songhurst & Kay Barnham
Researchers: David Bradbury & Sian Lewis
Senior Editor: Nicola Wright
Editorial Director: Colin Shelbourn
Design Manager: Kate Buxton
Assistant Designer: Deborah Chadwick
Production: Zoë Fawcett
Series Concept: Tony Potter

Colour separations by ScanTrans, Singapore
Printed by New Interlitho, Italy

First published in 1994 by Zigzag Publishing Ltd

Copyright © 1994 Zigzag Publishing Ltd

ISBN 1-85993-025-5

10 9 8 7 6 5 4 3 2 1

This book is about an amazing subject - you! It is packed full of fascinating information and facts about your body.

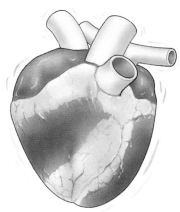

Discover why your blood is red and what you are made from. Find out how your brain works and how you digest food. These and many other fascinating topics are explored in clear text and colourful illustrations.

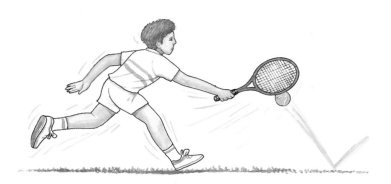

The illustrated timeline that runs through the book shows you the progress of medicine from earliest times to the present day. It lists important people, events, discoveries and inventions.

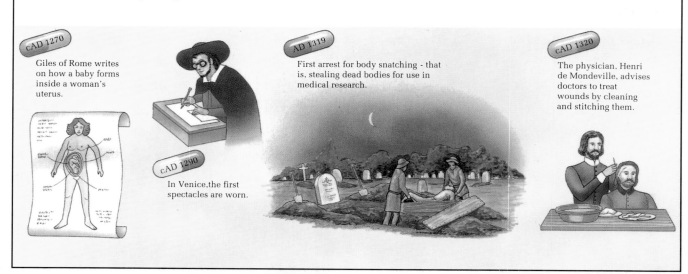

cAD 1270
Giles of Rome writes on how a baby forms inside a woman's uterus.

cAD 1290
In Venice, the first spectacles are worn.

AD 1319
First arrest for body snatching - that is, stealing dead bodies for use in medical research.

cAD 1320
The physician, Henri de Mondeville, advises doctors to treat wounds by cleaning and stitching them.

Contents

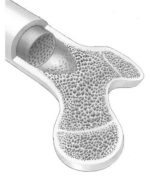
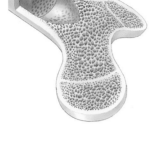
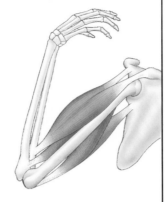
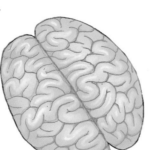
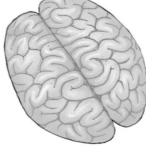
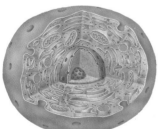
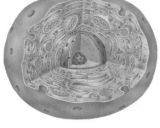
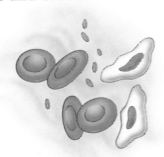
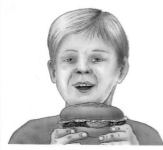
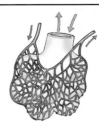
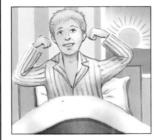
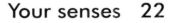
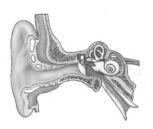
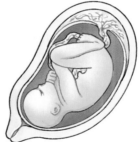
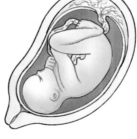
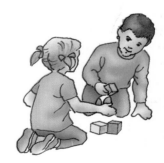
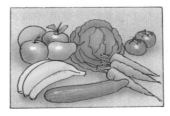
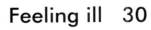
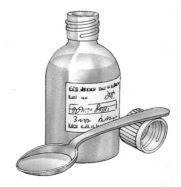

Why do we have bones?

If there were no bones in your body you would be like a floppy sack. You wouldn't be able to sit or stand, breathe or talk.

Marrow

Compact bone

Spongy bone

Are bones solid?

Bones are not hard all the way through. They are more like strong tubes. The outer layer is made of hard compact bone. Inside is a layer of spongy bone that looks like honeycomb. Some bones are filled with jelly-like red marrow. This is where most of the body's red blood cells are made.

Bone marrow makes 200 million new red blood cells every day!

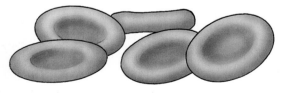

Moving

A joint is the place where two bones meet. Some joints, called hinge joints, work like door hinges and only bend in one direction.

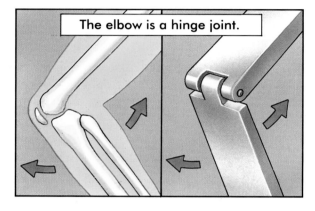

The elbow is a hinge joint.

Other joints are called ball and socket joints. The round end of one bone is able to move around in the hole formed by the other bone.

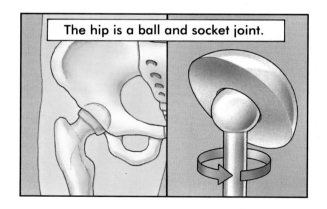

The hip is a ball and socket joint.

In some joints there is a fluid between the bones which helps them to work smoothly and move without rubbing against each other.

Big and small

All grown-ups have 206 different bones. The biggest is the thigh bone, and the smallest is the tiny stirrup bone inside each ear.

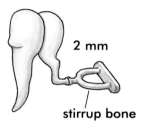

2 mm

stirrup bone

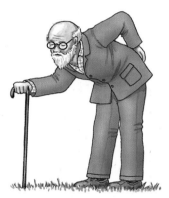

Old bones

Bones are very tough but, as people grow old, the joints between the bones can wear out. Sometimes, they become so worn that they will hardly move at all. This also happens to people who have the disease arthritis.

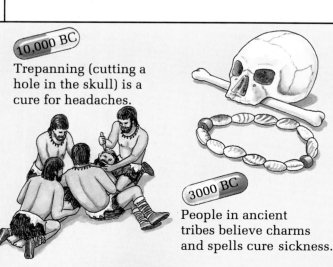

10,000 BC

Trepanning (cutting a hole in the skull) is a cure for headaches.

3000 BC

People in ancient tribes believe charms and spells cure sickness.

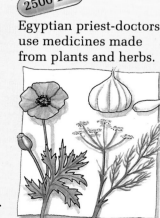

2500 BC

Egyptian priest-doctors use medicines made from plants and herbs.

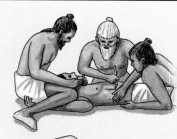

1500 BC

Surgeons in India carry out operations using saws, scissors, needles and forceps.

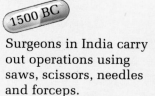

1000 BC

Acupuncture is used in China to treat the sick.

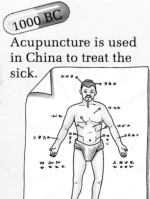

Ready to grow

Your bones have stopped growing before the age of about 20, unless you break one. Then new bones grows from both sides of the break until the pieces join back up again.

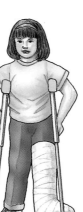

Light work

Bones need to be strong to hold you up and protect your body. The material they are made from is almost as strong as cast iron. Although they are strong, your bones do not weigh much. The total weight of an adult's bones is about 9 kg - the size of a medium sack of potatoes.

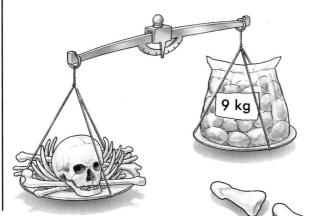

9 kg

Shrinking

By evening you are up to 1 cm shorter than you were in the morning! While you sleep, your body stretches out again to its full length. What happens is that the soft cushions of cartilage between the bones of your spine are squeezed down by your weight during the day and become squashed.

Is there a bone in your nose?

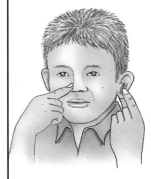

The hard part of your nose isn't a bone at all. It is a rubbery material called cartilage. The outer parts of your ears are made of cartilage too.

Bone count

Can you count the bones in your hand? You can feel the bones in your fingers and you can feel a few more in your palms.

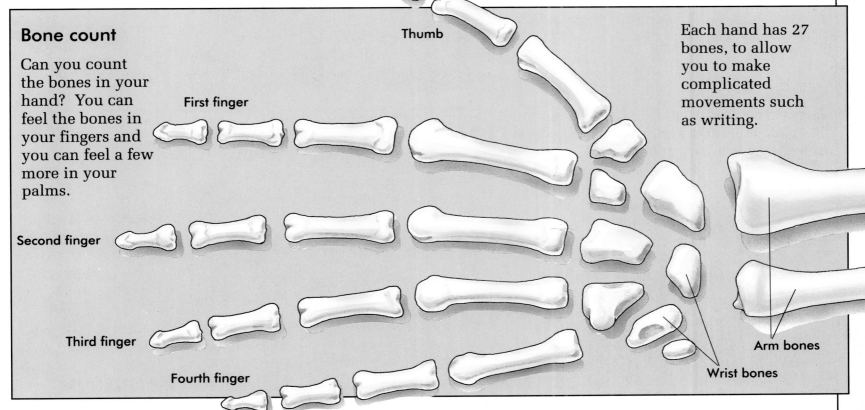

Thumb

First finger

Second finger

Third finger

Fourth finger

Each hand has 27 bones, to allow you to make complicated movements such as writing.

Arm bones

Wrist bones

600 BC
The Ancient Romans build sewage systems and public baths.

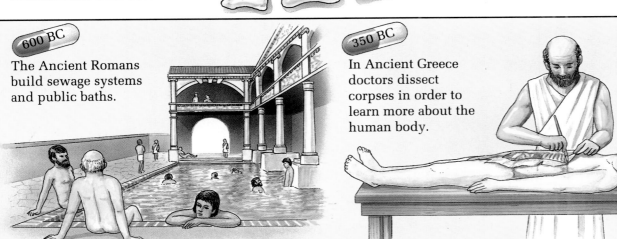

350 BC
In Ancient Greece doctors dissect corpses in order to learn more about the human body.

360 BC
Pupils of Greek physician Hippocrates learn that illness is not sent by the gods. They promise to help and never to harm the sick.

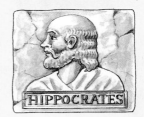

HIPPOCRATES

The way we move

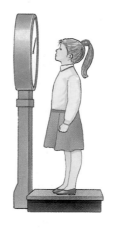

Neck muscles

Chest muscles

Biceps muscles

Thigh muscles

Calf muscles

Some of the main muscles in the body

Human beings use muscles with every move they make. Without muscles, you wouldn't be able to walk, run or even blink your eyes.

Lots of muscle

There are over 650 muscles in your body. That's three times the number of bones! In all, almost half your weight is muscles!

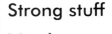

A big smile

Muscles in your tongue allow you to speak and eat and muscles in your eyes make them focus. When you walk, you use up to 200 muscles. It takes about 17 muscles to smile.

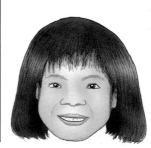

Strong stuff

Muscles are made up of bundles of long fibres. A muscle's power depends on how many fibres it has. The more exercise a muscle gets, the bigger and stronger the fibres grow. When they get no exercise, the fibres shrink and muscles grow weak.

Never tires

There is one muscle in your body that never gets tired, no matter how hard it works.

The heart is different from every other muscle. It beats over 100,000 times a day, pumping blood to every part of the body. If it stopped, you would die within a few minutes.

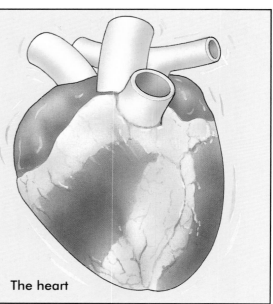

The heart

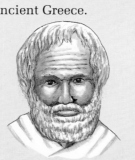
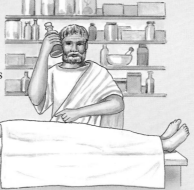
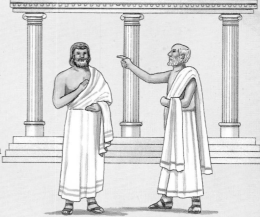

What are tendons?

Muscles are not joined straight on to bones. They are attached by strong, stretchy bands called tendons.

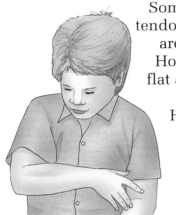

Some of the longest tendons in your body are in your hands. Hold one hand out flat and wiggle your little finger. Halfway up your arm a muscle will move. It is attached to your finger by a long tendon.

Are muscles all alike?

Different parts of the body have different kinds of muscle. Voluntary muscles move your arms, legs and head. You can control what they do.

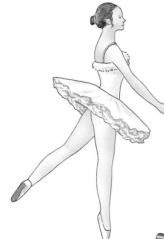

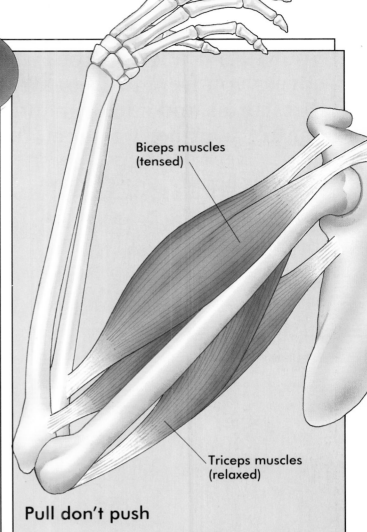

Biceps muscles (tensed)

Triceps muscles (relaxed)

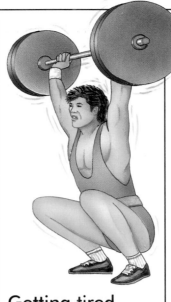

Getting tired

When a muscle is working hard it uses up lots of energy. It also gives out lots of heat and waste, called lactic acid. If the lactic acid builds up before the blood can carry it away the muscle gets tired. It slows down and becomes weaker.

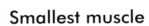

Involuntary muscles look after your breathing, the way you digest food and your heartbeat. You cannot make them stop or start, which is why it is impossible for you ever to forget to breathe

Smallest muscle

Your smallest muscle is in your ear. It is less than 3 mm long - about the size of a pencil point.

Pull don't push

Muscles only work by pulling, never by pushing. They can pull in just one direction - by making themselves shorter. The only way they can stretch out again is if another muscle pulls them back.

This is why many muscles work in pairs. Your arm is a good example. The biceps muscle pulls your arm up and bends the elbow. The triceps muscle, which pulls in the other direction, straightens out your arm again.

While the first muscle tenses up and pulls, the other one relaxes. Then the second pulls the other way, and the first one relaxes.

c100 BC

The Chinese describe how blood travels around the human body. In Europe, this is not discovered for another 700 years.

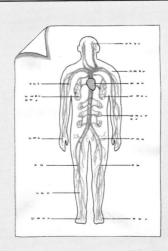

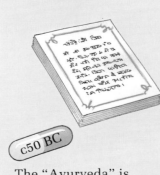

c50 BC

The "Ayurveda" is written. This is a Hindu medical book.

c.AD130

Greek physician Galen is born. Throughout his life, he collects medical information and writes the most important medical book for the next 1,500 years. He is the first doctor to measure pulse rate to find out what is wrong with a person.

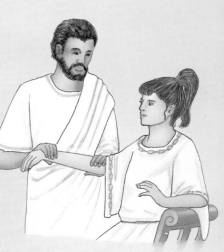

Outer wrapping

Your skin is a waterproof wrapping that covers you from head to toe. It keeps out dirt, germs and sunlight and helps to control your body temperature.

Double wrapped

Skin has two main layers. The tough, outer layer is called the epidermis. It is replaced all the time by new skin cells that grow underneath it.

As the old skin cells die, they harden and are rubbed away. Most of the dust you find in your home is made up of old, dead skin cells!

The inner layer of skin is called the dermis. It is much thicker than the epidermis. It is packed with nerve endings, hair roots, sweat glands and tiny blood vessels.

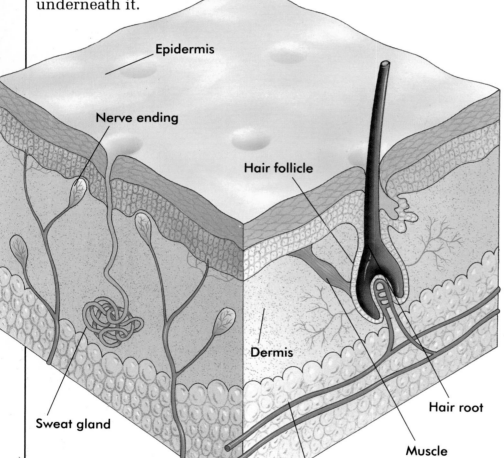

Epidermis

Nerve ending

Hair follicle

Dermis

Sweat gland

Hair root

Muscle

Blood vessel

Thick and thin

Most of your body is covered by a layer of skin 2 mm thick. But on the eyelids the skin is only about 0.5 mm thick, and on the soles of your feet the skin is as thick as 5 mm.

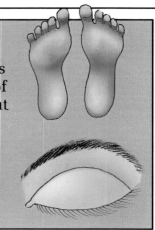

Goose bumps

When you get cold, hundreds of goose bumps form on your skin. At the root of every hair is a tiny muscle. When you are cold the muscle shrinks and pulls on the hair, making it stand up. This is the goose bump you see.

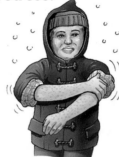

The hairs trap your body heat next to the skin. Animals with thick fur trap lots of air this way. Their fur works a bit like a duvet and helps keep them warm.

Black and blue

A bruise appears on your skin when you bump yourself hard. It starts when tiny blood vessels under the skin break and bleed. After a while the bruise turns black and blue. As it heals it turns yellow. Finally it fades away.

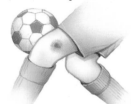

Freckles

Dark freckles appear where small patches of skin have produced extra melanin. People with pale skin are more likely to get freckles than those with dark skin.

AD 500s

The writings of Galen and Hippocrates are studied in European monasteries.

AD 540

Bubonic plague spreads across Europe and the Byzantine Empire. At its worst, 10,000 people die daily in the capital city, Constantinople.

AD 600s

In Europe, hospitals run by the Christian Church are set up to care for sick, mostly poor people.

AD 1000

The famous Medical School at Salerno, Italy, attracts students from all over the world.

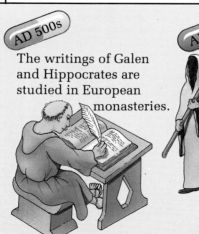
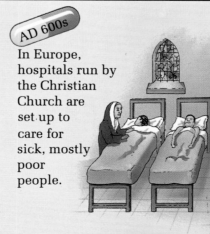
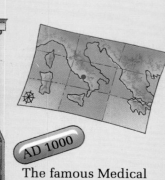

Clots and scabs

If you cut yourself, blood flows and soon makes a clot over the wound. It forms a thick, dark scab that protects the broken skin.

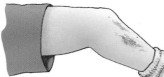

Meanwhile, new skin grows underneath at about 1 mm every two days. That is why you must not pick at scabs! Once the skin has healed, the scab falls off.

Keeping cool

When you get very hot you sweat. Sweating is a way your body cools itself. Tiny sweat glands in your skin leak salty water through holes called pores. As the water dries it cools your skin down.

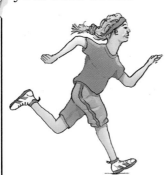

Fingerprints

Your fingertips are covered with a pattern of tiny ridges. No two people in the world have the same pattern.

Fingerprints can help solve crimes. A fingerprint found at the scene of a crime may match prints that are already on police files.

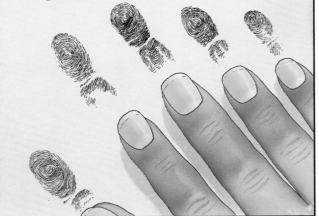

Hair raising

Hair grows out of pits in the skin called follicles. Each hair grows about 1 cm a month from the root at the bottom of the follicle. As the hair grows it dies and hardens. That is why it doesn't hurt to have your hair cut.

Each hair lives for about two or three years. Then it falls out. In time, a new one starts to grow in its place. Every day, you lose about 50-100 hairs.

People with red hair have around 90,000 hairs on their heads. Blondes have around 140,000 hairs. People with black or brown hair have about 110,000 hairs.

Straight, wavy, curly

The shape of your hair follicles also shapes your hair. Round follicles make straight hair. Oval follicles make wavy hair. Flat follicles produce curly hair.

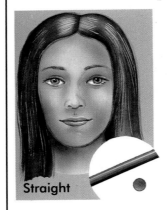

Straight

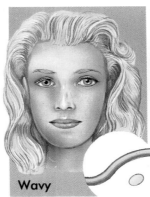

Wavy

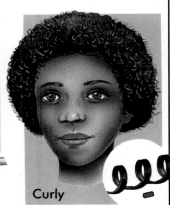

Curly

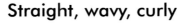

AD 1009

The *Canon of Medicine* is written by Avicenna, a Persian physician. This set of 5 books about Greek and Arabic medicine is used in Europe to teach medicine until the 1800s.

AD 1100s

The *Rule of Health* is published by the School of Salerno. It includes advice on treating illness, on diet, cleanliness and good health.

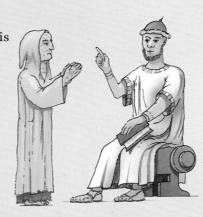

AD 1140

The Norman king, Roger II, declares that physicians cannot work without an official government permit.

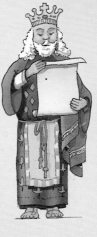

Brain power

Your brain is the most important organ you have. It never stops working even while you are asleep. It is busy all the time, receiving information and sending out instructions to every part of your body.

Like a walnut

Inside your skull is something that looks like a huge walnut. This is your brain. Like a walnut, it has two halves - the left brain and the right.

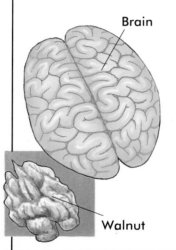

Brain

Walnut

Millions of cells

The brain is made of millions of tiny nerve cells, called neurons. There are long neurons that carry messages to and from your body and short neurons that link together different areas in the brain.

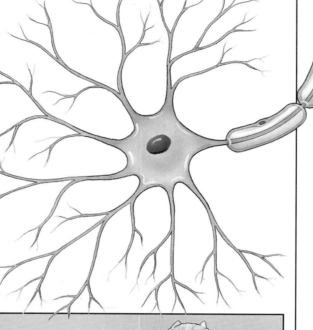

Control centres

Different areas of the cortex have different jobs to do. One area controls your thoughts and feelings, another deals with speech, and yet another with movement.

Cerebrum (biggest part of the brain) and the cortex (its surface)

Three parts

The brain is divided into three main parts. The largest is the cerebrum. Its crinkly surface, called the cortex, is packed into thousands of folds and loops. Stretched out, the cortex would be about the size of a pillow case (about 3,000 sq cm).

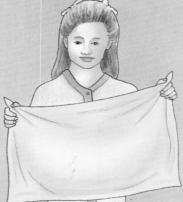

Balance

The part of the brain called the cerebellum helps the cortex to control complex movements, such as walking or writing. This area also controls balance.

cAD 1270

Giles of Rome writes on how a baby forms inside a woman's uterus.

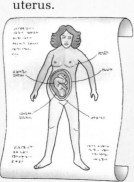

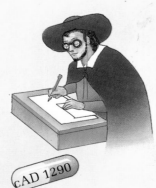

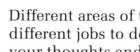
AD 1319

First arrest for body snatching - that is, stealing dead bodies for use in medical research.

cAD 1320

The physician, Henri de Mondeville, advises doctors to treat wounds by cleaning and stitching them.

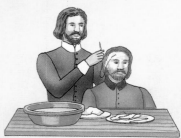

cAD 1290

In Venice, the first spectacles are worn.

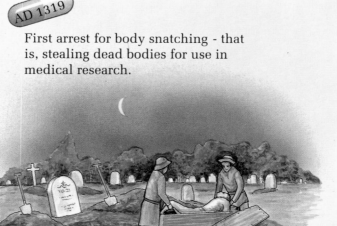

Left or right?

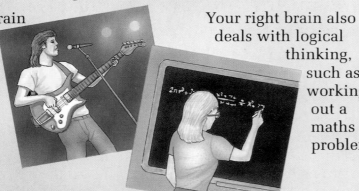

The left brain and the right brain are joined by a thick bundle of nerves. It may seem strange, but the left brain controls the right side of your body, and the right brain controls the left!

Your left brain also controls creative talents, such as musical skills.

Your right brain also deals with logical thinking, such as working out a maths problem.

Nervous system

A thick bundle of nerves runs down from the brain stem to the spinal cord, which is inside your backbone. Smaller bundles of nerves branch out from the spinal cord and reach to every part of the body.

The brain and spinal cord make up your central nervous system

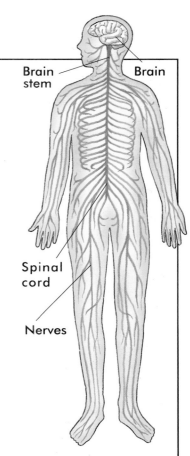

Brain stem

Brain

Spinal cord

Nerves

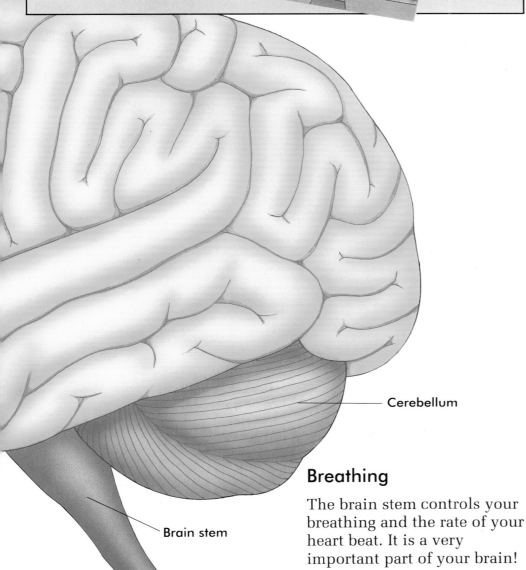

Cerebellum

Brain stem

Breathing

The brain stem controls your breathing and the rate of your heart beat. It is a very important part of your brain!

Electrical signals

Signals travel from different parts of the body to the brain along the nerves. They carry these messages in the form of tiny, electrical impulses.

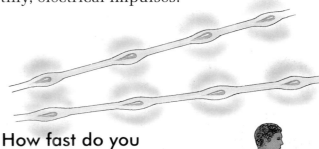

How fast do you think?

Your nerves can carry messages at speeds of up to 460 km/h. That is fast enough to travel the length of a football field in half a second!

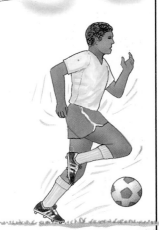

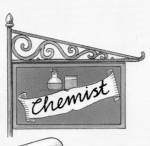

AD 1345

The first chemist's shop opens in London.

cAD 1350

The Black Death sweeps across Europe. This incurable plague kills thousands of people.

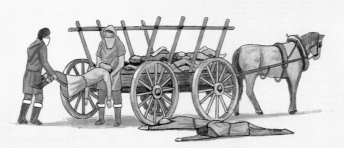

cAD 1360

A paper is published on mending bones.

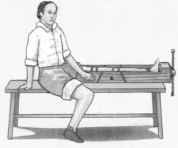

AD 1377

A quarantine centre opens at Ragusa, Yugoslavia. Anyone with plague symptoms must stay there for forty days.

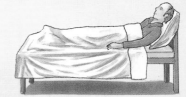

Super cells

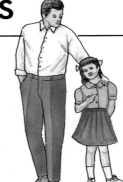

All human beings are made of tiny, separate parts called cells. They are so small that you can only see them with a powerful microscope.

Big people

The bigger a person is, the more cells he or she has. Children do not have as many cells as adults, but they have the same kinds.

Cell count

Adults have about 50 billion cells in their bodies, and there are over a hundred different kinds!

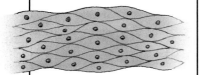

Each kind groups together to make different sorts of body material, or tissue, such as muscle, bone or blood.

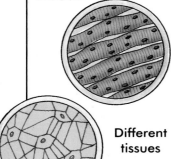

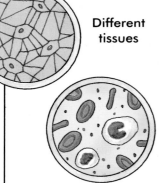

Different tissues

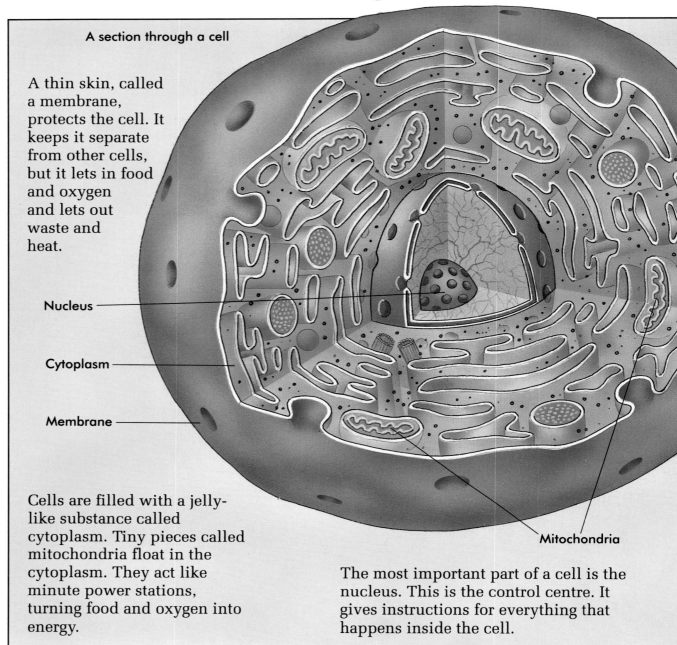

A section through a cell

A thin skin, called a membrane, protects the cell. It keeps it separate from other cells, but it lets in food and oxygen and lets out waste and heat.

Nucleus

Cytoplasm

Membrane

Mitochondria

Cells are filled with a jelly-like substance called cytoplasm. Tiny pieces called mitochondria float in the cytoplasm. They act like minute power stations, turning food and oxygen into energy.

The most important part of a cell is the nucleus. This is the control centre. It gives instructions for everything that happens inside the cell.

AD 1403

Bethlehem Royal Hospital in London becomes a lunatic asylum. The inmates are not treated.

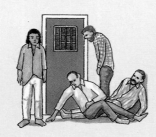

AD 1493

Explorers in America discover that the native American Indians there use tobacco as a medicine. They also smoke it.

AD 1500

The first Caesarian operation on a living woman is performed by a Swiss pig-farmer on his wife.

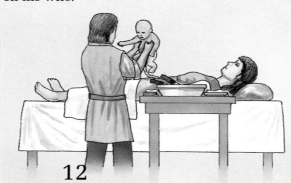

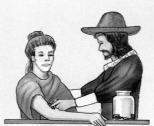

AD 1500

Blood-letting is a common treatment for illnesses.

Central heating

All cells take in food and oxygen and give out heat and waste. As the food and oxygen gets used up inside the cell, it provides you with energy and heats up your body. When you exercise hard, the cells make heat and energy up to 40 times faster!

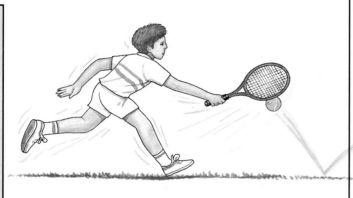

Starting life

No matter how big or small they are, all human beings start life as a single cell that divides over and over again and grows into a baby inside its mother's body.

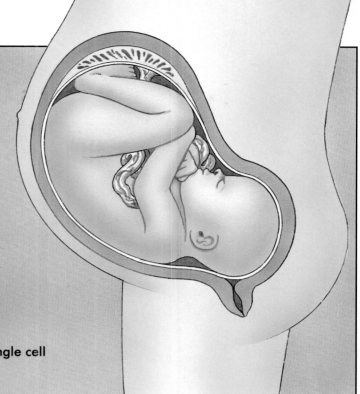

 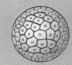

A baby grows from a single cell

Big and small

The biggest cells are the female's egg cells, called ova. You can just about see them with the naked eye.

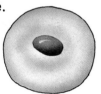

Brain cells are the smallest cells in the body.

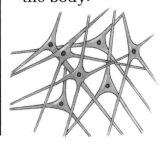

New cells

Every day, millions of body cells die and millions more take their place. You lose thousands of brain cells daily! A new cell is made when an existing cell grows and divides in two. The new cell is an exact copy of the old one.

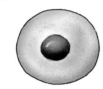

Single cell

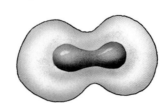

Nucleus dividing

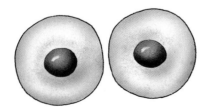

Two new cells

Funny shapes

Different cells are different shapes. Nerve cells are very long. They have branch-like fibres attached to them, for passing messages around the body.

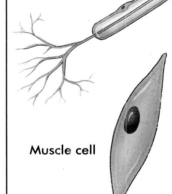

Nerve cell

Sperm cell

Muscle cell

Muscle cells are shaped like tiny tubes, while male sperm cells have long, whip-like tails to help them move fast.

AD 1518

The Royal College of Physicians is founded in London by a charter granted by Henry VIII.

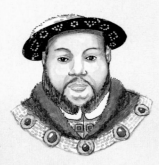

AD 1529

Dissections of corpses are carried out at Padua University in Italy.

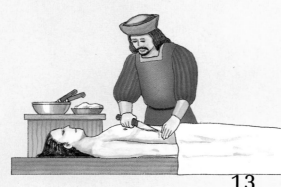

AD 1540

Wooden limbs are fitted to soldiers who have lost arms or legs in battle.

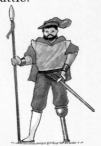

AD 1545

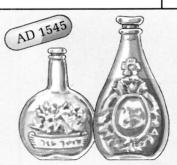

Soothing ointments are used to treat wounds instead of boiling oil!

What is blood?

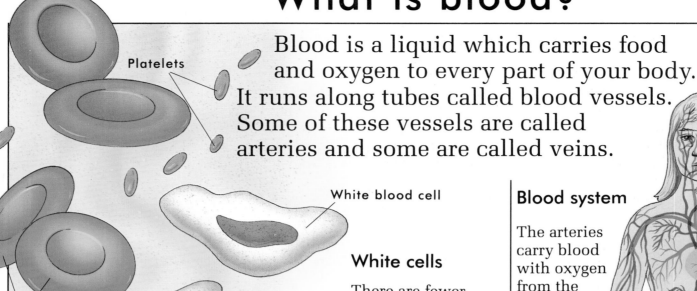

Blood is a liquid which carries food and oxygen to every part of your body. It runs along tubes called blood vessels. Some of these vessels are called arteries and some are called veins.

Platelets

White blood cell

Red blood cells

Plasma is 90% water

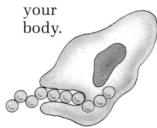

What is blood made of?

Blood is made up of red blood cells, white blood cells and platelets. These float in a yellowish liquid called plasma.

Red blood

The blood in your arteries is rich in oxygen and so it is bright red. Can you see the veins along your arms? They have very little oxygen - they probably look purple or blue!

White cells

There are fewer white blood cells than red ones. White cells are the army of your blood system! They hunt down and kill any harmful bacteria or viruses in your body.

Blood system

heart

The arteries carry blood with oxygen from the heart to every part of the body.

The veins carry blood with waste (especially carbon dioxide) to the heart and lungs where it receives fresh oxygen.

The arteries are in red and the veins are in blue.

The arteries and veins divide many times. They lead into tiny, hollow thread-like blood vessels called capillaries.

How platelets help cuts to heal

If you have an accident and cut your skin, blood flows out. This cleans the wound. The tiny blood platelets start to stick together. They make a plug over the cut. The blood hardens into a scab. New skin cells start to grow underneath the scab, which eventually falls off.

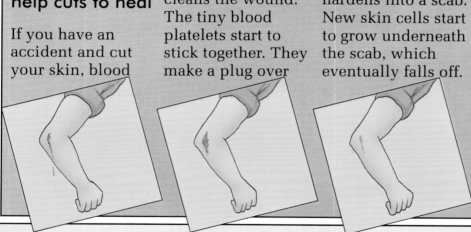

AD 1542

Surgeon, Andreas Versalis, describes the workings of the human body in a book

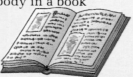

illustrated with hundreds of detailed drawings.

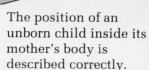
AD 1559

The position of an unborn child inside its mother's body is described correctly.

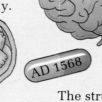

AD 1568

The structure of the human brain is properly described.

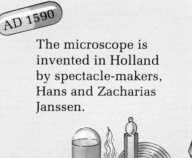
AD 1590

The microscope is invented in Holland by spectacle-makers, Hans and Zacharias Janssen.

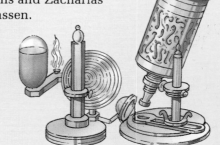

Clean blood

To keep your blood really clean and healthy, about 250 million new blood

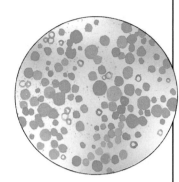

cells are made every day in your bone marrow.

World record!

If all your arteries and veins were laid out from end to end, they would stretch 100,000 km. That is two and a half times around the world!

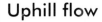

Uphill flow

Special flaps, called valves, in the heart, arteries and veins stop the blood from flowing backwards, even when it is sent uphill.

Blood types

People have different types of blood. There are four main types: A, B, AB and O. If you lose a lot of blood, it needs to be replaced in a blood transfusion. Doctors test your blood to see what type it is. If blood from certain groups is mixed together you can become very ill.

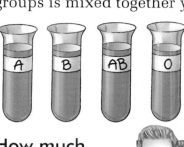

How much blood?

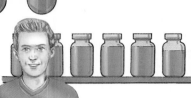

An adult's body contains about 6 litres of blood.

The heart

Your heart is about the size of a fist. It has two sides. The right-hand side takes in blood from the veins. It pumps the blood to the lungs where it receives oxygen. From the lungs, the blood travels to the left-hand side of the heart. From here, it is pumped along the arteries to every part of the body.

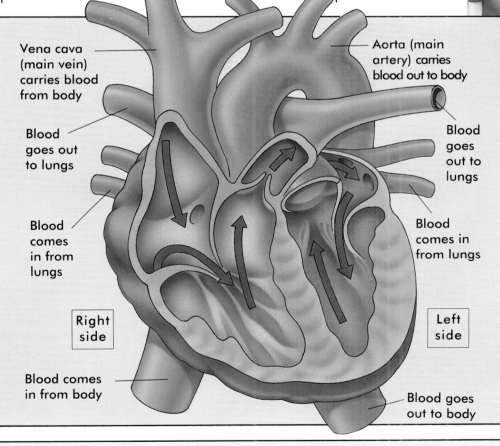

Vena cava (main vein) carries blood from body

Aorta (main artery) carries blood out to body

Blood goes out to lungs

Blood comes in from lungs

Blood goes out to lungs

Blood comes in from lungs

Right side

Left side

Blood comes in from body

Blood goes out to body

Your heart never stops beating. It tightens and relaxes about 70 to 80 times a minute. This rhythm works as a pump, pushing the blood around your body.

Your heart is so powerful that it only takes one minute for each blood cell to travel all round your body and back to your heart!

The scientist Galileo invents the first thermometer. It is a glass tube filled with coloured water.

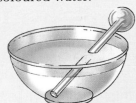

Sweat gland

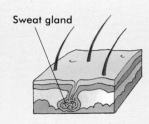

The way in which human beings sweat is first studied and described.

Thomas Sydenham of England describes measles and identifies scarlet fever.

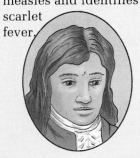

William Harvey describes how blood flows around the body.

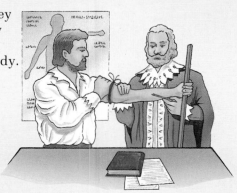

Eating and digesting

Food is the fuel your body needs to keep it alive and working. The food you eat is digested (broken down into tiny pieces) inside your body and sent to all your cells.

From start to finish

Food starts to be digested in your mouth. Next, it travels down the oesophagus (food pipe) into the stomach. In the small intestine, more digestion takes place. Undigested food goes in to the large intestine before passing out of the body through the rectum.

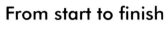

Mouth

Oesophagus

Stomach

Large intestine

Rectum

Small intestine

Inside the stomach

Gastric juices, made in the stomach wall, mix with the food and break it down. The stomach walls squeeze and mix the food. Acid in the juices also kills any germs.

The lining of the stomach wall makes a special mucus that keeps the food wet, and also stops the stomach from digesting itself!

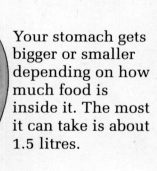

Your stomach gets bigger or smaller depending on how much food is inside it. The most it can take is about 1.5 litres.

AD 1639

A medicine called quinine made from tree bark is used to treat malaria and other tropical fevers.

AD 1658

Sir Thomas Browne, an English doctor, recommends cremating dead bodies rather than burying them.

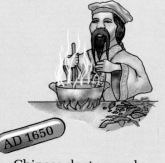
AD 1650

Chinese doctors make medicines by boiling up herbs to make special infusions.

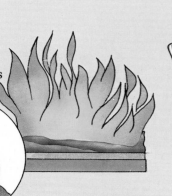

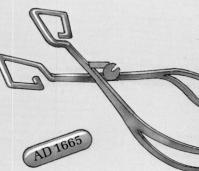
AD 1665

Forceps are invented to help with the delivery of babies.

The small intestine

Inside the small intestine, the food is mixed with more juices, breaking it down even further.

The finger-like villi that line the small intestine have blood vessels inside them.

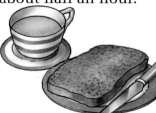

When the food has broken down enough, tiny food substances called nutrients pass through the intestine wall. The nutrients go into the blood stream. They are carried all round the body to provide fuel for the cells.

After up to 3 hours in the stomach the food is like thick soup. It is now sent, a little at a time, into the small intestine.

Biggest part

The small intestine is the biggest part of your digestive system! It is very narrow - only about 2.5 cm in diameter, but in adults it is about 6 metres long!

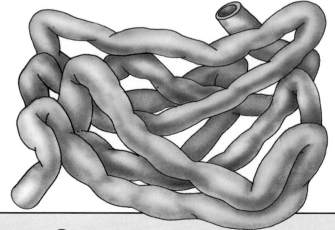

Hard to digest

Food is made up of proteins, carbohydrates, and fats. Proteins are the hardest to digest. A low-protein meal of tea and toast stays in your stomach for about half an hour.

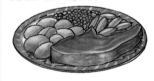

A high-protein meal of meat and vegetables might stay in your stomach for up to four hours!

The large intestine

Water and food which cannot be digested are now sent to the large intestine. It is much thicker than the small intestine, but only about 1.5 metres long.

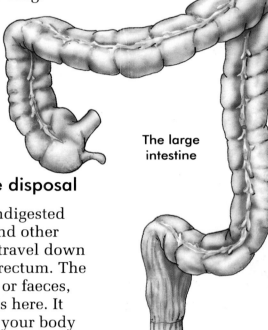

The large intestine

Waste disposal

The undigested food and other waste travel down to the rectum. The waste, or faeces, collects here. It leaves your body through an opening called the anus.

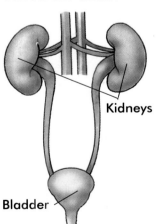

Kidneys

Bladder

Long wait

Food stays in the large intestine for up to 20 hours. Water passes into the blood stream. It is taken, with other waste material, to the kidneys.

The bladder

Your bladder is a strong bag of muscle. Urine (waste fluid) is sent here from the kidneys. The full bladder empties in to a tube called the urethra that leads out of your body.

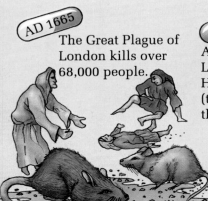

AD 1665
The Great Plague of London kills over 68,000 people.

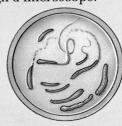

AD 1676
Antony van Leeuwenhoek of Holland sees microbes (tiny forms of life) through a microscope.

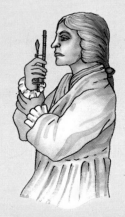

AD 1736
First successful operation for appendicitis is carried out.

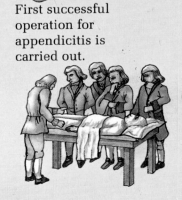

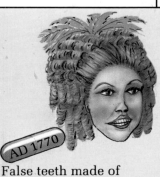

AD 1770
False teeth made of porcelain are fitted to patients in France. They are the first comfortable dentures.

All about breathing

All living things must breathe to stay alive. When you breathe, air goes into your lungs. The lungs take out the oxygen from the air. Your blood then carries the oxygen to all the cells in your body.

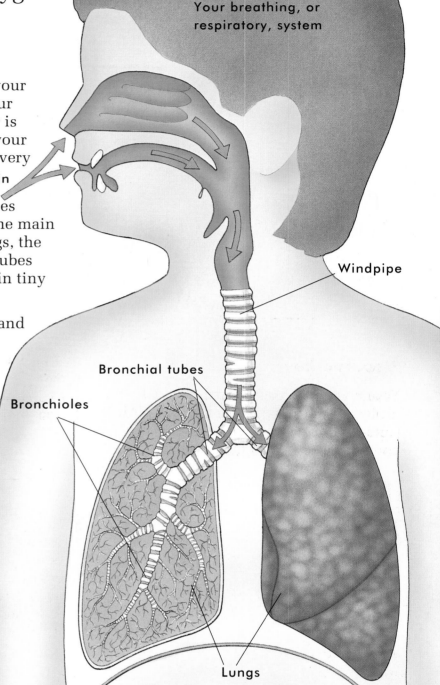

Your breathing, or respiratory, system

Air goes in

Windpipe

Bronchial tubes

Bronchioles

Lungs

Into the bloodstream

When you breathe in, the millions of alveoli in your lungs fill with air. Tiny blood vessels around the alveoli take in the oxygen from the air. It is then carried all round your body.

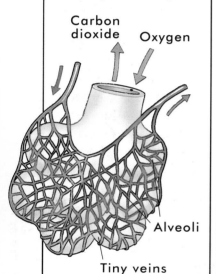

Carbon dioxide

Oxygen

Alveoli

Tiny veins

The alveoli also take back carbon dioxide from the blood vessels. This waste gas leaves your body when you breathe out.

How air gets in

Air gets in to your body through your mouth or nose. It is sent down your windpipe into your lungs. The air is warmed by tiny blood vessels in your windpipe. Your lungs do not like very cold air!

Your windpipe splits into two tubes called bronchial tubes. There is one main tube for each lung. Inside the lungs, the tubes split up into many smaller tubes called bronchioles which end up in tiny air sacs called alveoli.

Your lungs are very light, spongy and stretchy. They spring back into shape as you breathe in and out.

High places

The higher you go, the less oxygen there is in the air. People from mountainous places have larger lungs than normal. They need to breathe in more air at a time to get the right amount of oxygen.

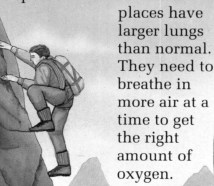

 AD 1792

The first ambulance specially made to carry wounded people is built. It is pulled by horses.

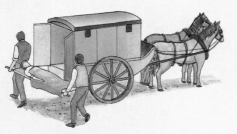

 AD 1796

Edward Jenner begins to use vaccination as a way of protecting people against the disease smallpox.

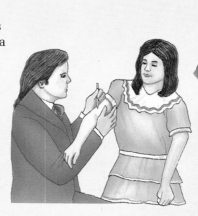

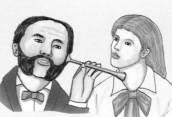

 AD 1816

The stethoscope is first used. It has one earpiece. Modern, two earpiece types appear in 1850.

AD 1823

The respected medical journal *The Lancet* is first published.

THE LANCET

Breathing in

When you breathe in, a large flat muscle under your lungs (called the diaphragm) pushes down. Your ribs move up and out. Air is sucked down your windpipe and fills your lungs.

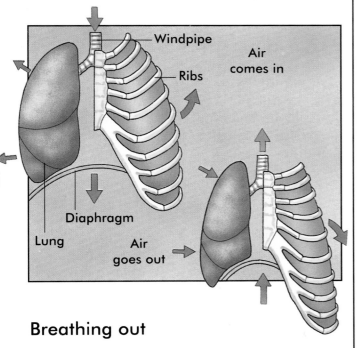

Windpipe

Air comes in

Ribs

Diaphragm

Lung

Air goes out

Breathing out

Your ribs move back and the muscle under your lungs springs up again. Air is squeezed out of your lungs. It goes up your windpipe and out of your mouth.

Talking

You cannot talk without air! Sounds are made when air is pushed past the two vocal cords in your larynx, or voice box. As the air from your lungs pushes past, the vocal cords vibrate.

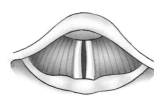

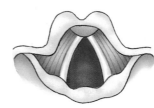

Top: the vocal cords are closed

Below: air from the lungs pushes past the vocal cords

The wrong tube!

Your windpipe is next to your food pipe. When you swallow, a special flap at the top of your throat (called the epiglottis) covers the opening to the windpipe to stop any food going down the wrong way!

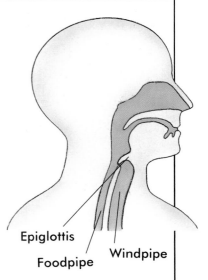

Epiglottis

Foodpipe   Windpipe

Hiccups

You get hiccups when your diaphragm moves jerkily. This makes you take in short, quick breaths of air. The funny hiccup noise is made by the vocal cords as they open and close with the sudden rushes of air.

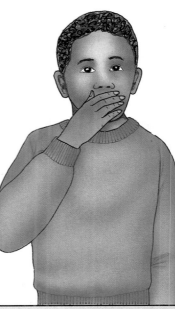

How much air?

Take a deep breath. How much air can you take in? Adults can hold as much as 6 litres of air in their lungs!

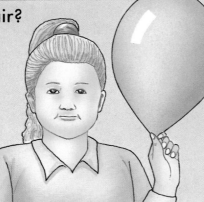

Normally, people hold about 2.5 litres of air in their lungs all the time.

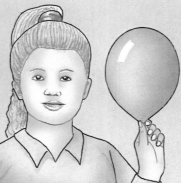

They take in and breathe out about 0.5 litres of air at a time.

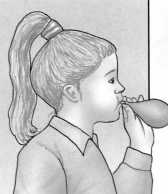

AD 1825

A blood transfusion is made from one person to another.

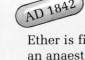
AD 1842

Ether is first used as an anaesthetic to send patients to sleep so that they feel no pain during an operation.

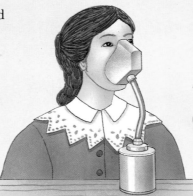

AD 1851

The first opthalmoscope is used to examine the back of the eye.

AD 1852

Plaster-soaked bandages are used to set broken bones.

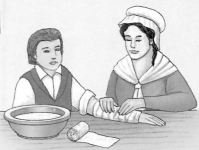

Why you need sleep

Did you know that you spend about one-third of your life asleep? While you sleep, you rest more than at any other time. Your body does not waste sleeping time - it has plenty to do while you are snoozing.

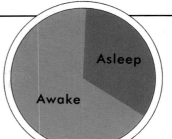

Asleep

Awake

Brain activity

Your brain is still busy at night. It sends messages to make sure that you breathe and your heart beats regularly while you are asleep. In the morning, part of your brain (the thalamus and the pons) sends out a wake-up call!

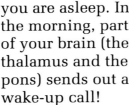

Cortex

Thalamus

Cerebellum   Pons

Brain stem

REM

Most people only remember their dreams if they wake during the dream or just afterwards. When we dream our eyes start to move. This is called Rapid Eye Movement (REM). After each REM period we fall into a deep sleep.

Heavenly messages

People used to think that dreams were messages sent from the gods. Today, we know that dreams are made up by our sleeping minds. They are often about things that have happened during the day.

Sweet dreams

We dream about one quarter of the time we are asleep, yet scientists still do not know exactly why we do it!

Cooling down

When you sleep, your body's workings slow down. Your heart pumps blood around your body more slowly. This cools you down. For a good night's sleep, you should make sure that your duvet or blankets keep you warm enough.

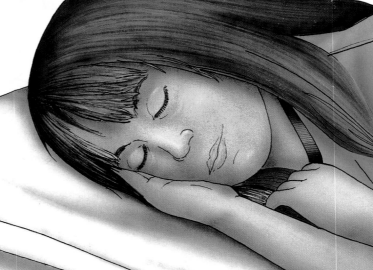

AD 1853

A hypodermic syringe is used for the first time to give a patient an injection under the skin.

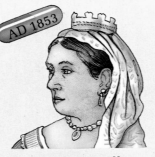

AD 1853

Queen Victoria allows herself to be treated with chloroform gas during the birth of her seventh child.

AD 1855

English nurse Florence Nightingale introduces proper nursing and hygiene to battlefield hospitals.

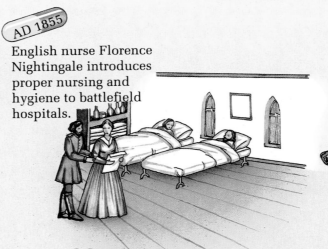

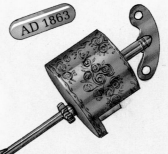

AD 1863

A simple kind of dental drill is invented that runs by clockwork.

Early to bed...

The amount of sleep you need depends on your age. When you are young, your body is growing and needs more sleep. A newborn baby can sleep for up to 20 hours a day.

At the age of four, children need 10-14 hours sleep. By the time you are nine, you might sleep for about 9 hours a night. Adults do not need as much sleep as children.

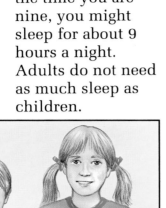

20 hours   14 hours   9 hours

Recharging your body

While you are asleep, the energy that your body has used during the day is built up again, so that you have plenty of energy the next morning. Special growth chemicals, called hormones, help your body to repair itself and grow.

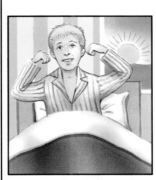

Sleepwalking

Some people walk or talk while they are asleep, especially if they are worried or anxious about something.

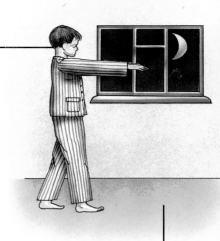

No sleep!

If they have no sleep at all for long periods of time, people get muddled up and lose their concentration. If you did not sleep for 10 days or more, you would go mad or even die!

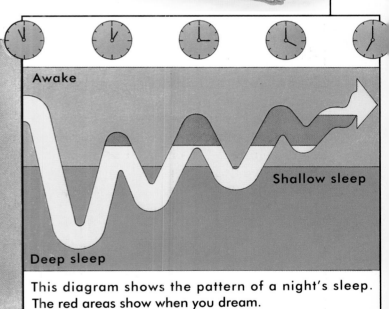

Awake

Shallow sleep

Deep sleep

This diagram shows the pattern of a night's sleep. The red areas show when you dream.

AD 1863

Doctors begin to use the mercury-filled thermometer.

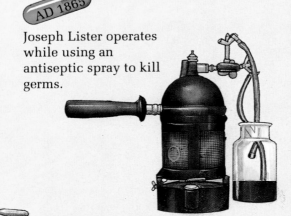
AD 1865

Joseph Lister operates while using an antiseptic spray to kill germs.

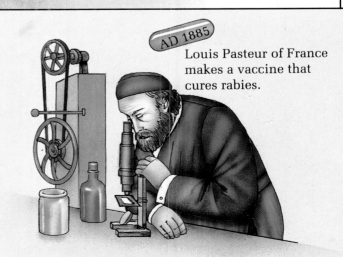
AD 1885

Louis Pasteur of France makes a vaccine that cures rabies.

Your senses

You have five senses: sight, hearing, smell, taste and touch. Special receptor cells in your body pick up information about the world around you and send it on to your brain.

How you see

Seeing is perhaps your most important sense. Your eyes work like very fast cameras.

Each eye is moved by six tiny muscles. The muscles move your eyes up, down, round and sideways!

Light rays

Pupil

Retina

Optic nerve

1. Rays of light enter your eyes through your pupils.

2. The lens can become fatter or thinner to make sure that a clear image lands on your retina.

3. The light rays cross over and an upside-down image forms on your retina, at the back of your eyeball.

4. Cells in the retina pick up the light rays. They send signals along the optic nerve to your brain.

5. Your brain turns the image the right way up.

Blue eyes?

You get your eye colour from your parents. If they both have blue eyes you will probably have blue eyes. But if one parent has brown eyes and one parent has blue eyes, their children will nearly always have brown eyes, as this is the stronger colour.

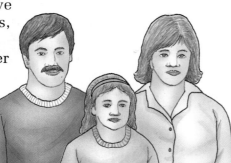

Your sense of touch

Your skin contains millions of nerve endings. These collect information and send messages to your brain. There are also about 500,000 special touch receptors. Most are in your tongue, lips and fingertips.

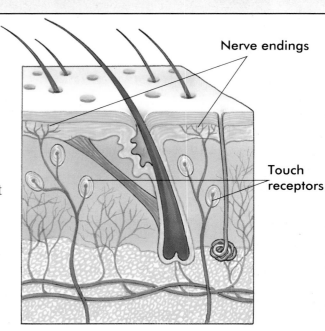

Nerve endings

Touch receptors

AD 1890

Rubber gloves are worn for the first time during surgery.

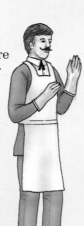

AD 1891

In Germany, chemotherapy is used to cure sick people. They are given drugs that kill the harmful bacteria in their bodies.

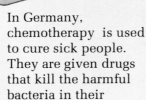

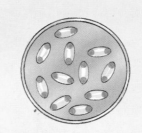

AD 1894

The bacteria that causes bubonic plague is discovered.

AD 1895

Wilhelm Röntgen discovers X-rays, which can be used for taking pictures of the bones inside people.

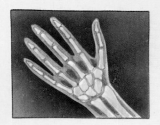

How you hear

Sounds are really vibrations in the air. Your ears collect the vibrations and funnel them in to the ear drum.

The vibrations reach the cochlea, which is lined with nerve endings that send messages to the brain.

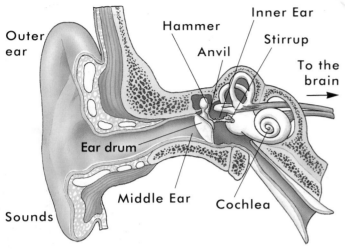

Outer ear

Hammer

Anvil

Inner Ear

Stirrup

To the brain

Ear drum

Middle Ear

Cochlea

Sounds

The ear drum shakes and passes the vibrations on to three small bones: the hammer, anvil and stirrup.

The brain translates the messages as sounds.

Sense of balance

The cochlea and the three loops above it are filled with liquid. The liquid moves when you do. Tiny nerve endings feel where the liquid in the loops is and pass on messages to your brain. Your brain then knows whether you are balanced or in danger of falling over!

The cochlea helps your sense of balance

Dizzy!

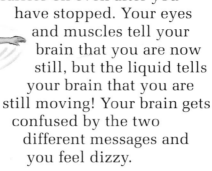

If you spin round, the liquid in your ears also spins. It carries on even after you have stopped. Your eyes and muscles tell your brain that you are now still, but the liquid tells your brain that you are still moving! Your brain gets confused by the two different messages and you feel dizzy.

Your sense of smell

Special smell receptors in your nose pick up information about smells. They send on the messages to your brain. Some smells are pleasant and inviting. Nasty smells warn you to stay away! The sense cells in your nose can tell the difference between thousands of kinds of smells.

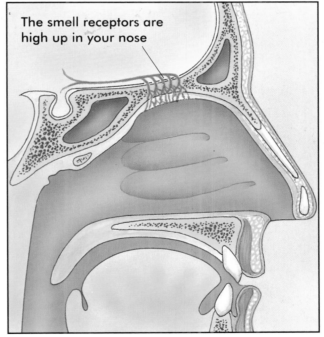
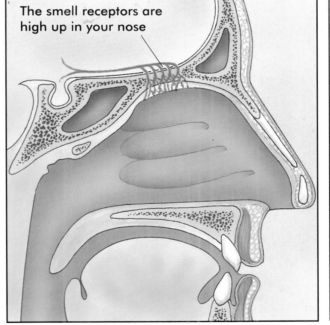

The smell receptors are high up in your nose

Your sense of taste

Tastebuds on your tongue send messages to your brain about what you are eating. There are four main tastes: bitter, sweet, salt and sour. Different parts of your tongue sense the different tastes.

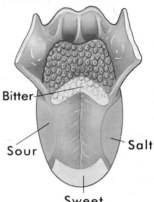

Bitter

Sour

Salt

Sweet

Bless you!

Food does not taste the same when you have a cold. This is because your sense of taste is closely linked to your sense of smell.

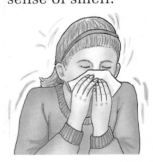

AD 1806

Blood pressure is measured using an inflatable rubber cuff on the arm and a measuring instrument called a sphygmomanometer.

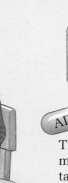

AD 1897

The drug aspirin is manufactured. When taken, aspirin lowers fever and stops aches and pains.

AD 1901

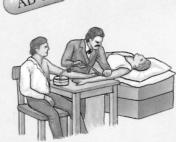

Blood groups A, B and O are discovered. People within the same groups can have safe blood transfusions.

AD 1902

The British Queen, Alexandra, is one of the first people to use an electrical hearing aid.

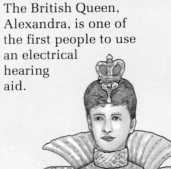

How babies are made

Each new life begins with just one cell. This cell is made when a male sperm enters a female egg.

Inside a woman's body

Each month, one of a woman's ovaries releases an egg, or ovum. It travels down one of the Fallopian tubes that lead into the uterus, or womb.

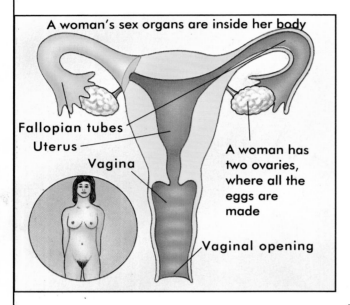

A woman's sex organs are inside her body

Fallopian tubes
Uterus
Vagina

A woman has two ovaries, where all the eggs are made

Vaginal opening

Making love

Sexual intercourse happens when a man and a woman love one another. It is often called making love. The man puts his penis inside the woman's vagina and millions of sperm shoot out of the end of his penis. The sperm swim towards the Fallopian tubes.

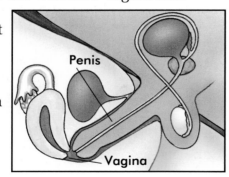

Penis

Vagina

Inside a man's body

Millions of sperm are made inside the man's testes. These are two organs inside a bag of loose skin close to the penis. During sexual intercourse, sperm travel along the tubes and out through the penis.

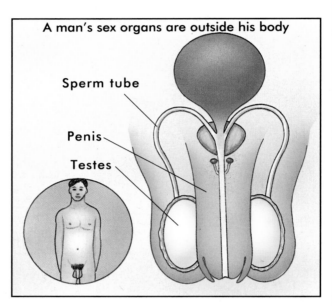

A man's sex organs are outside his body

Sperm tube

Penis

Testes

Sperm factory

The testes make 300 million new sperm every day! The sperm swim in a liquid called semen. If they are not released, the sperm die off and are absorbed into the body.

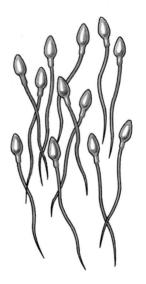

Sperm swim in semen

How life begins

A baby's life begins when an egg joins with a sperm. Only one sperm is able to enter the egg. This is called fertilization. It is the moment a baby is begun, or conceived.

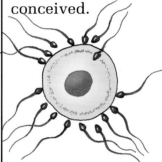

Each sperm has a tail to help it swim. After a sperm has wriggled inside an egg, its tail falls off.

Within a few hours the fertilized egg starts to divide. The ball of dividing cells travels to the uterus and attaches itself to the wall lining.

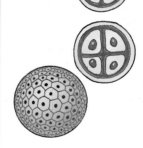

The Rorschach inkblot test is developed. Patients describe what images they see in inkblots.

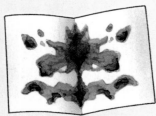

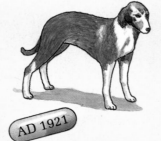

Experiments are made on dogs with the condition diabetes, using insulin taken from the human pancreas.

French scientists, Calmette and Guerin develop a vaccine against the disease tuberculosis.

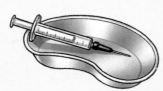

White blood cells are discovered.

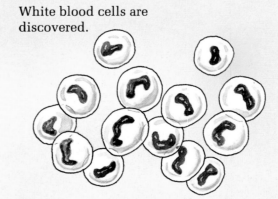

Countdown!

It takes about 38 weeks from fertilization for a baby to be ready to be born. During this time it grows rapidly.

4 weeks: The baby is about 0.6 cm long. Its heart begins to beat.

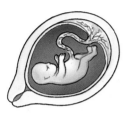

12 weeks: The baby is almost fully formed but only about 6-7 cm long.

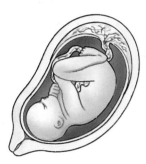

28 weeks: The baby is 30-36 cm long and weighs about 900 grams. If it was born now it would have a good chance of surviving.

Inside the uterus

Where the growing ball of cells attaches itself to the uterus wall a special organ, the placenta, forms. A long cord, the umbilical cord, joins the baby to the placenta.

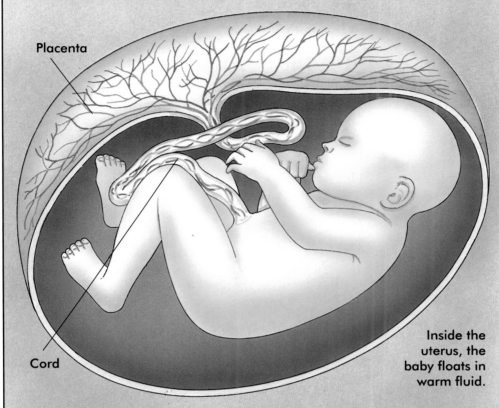

Placenta

Cord

Inside the uterus, the baby floats in warm fluid.

Food and oxygen from the mother's bloodstream enter the placenta and travel along the cord into the baby's body. Waste and carbon dioxide from the baby is carried back along the cord to the placenta.

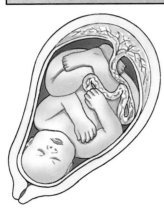

38 weeks: The baby is about 50 cm long and weighs about 3.5 kg. It is now ready to be born.

Girl or boy?

Every cell in the body contains 46 chromosomes. These contain all the information about the body's characteristics (like hair colour, size and weight).

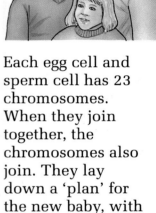

Each egg cell and sperm cell has 23 chromosomes. When they join together, the chromosomes also join. They lay down a 'plan' for the new baby, with characteristics from both parents, including whether it will be a boy or a girl!

Twins

Sometimes, two babies grow inside the mother at the same time. Identical twins are made when one fertilized egg splits into two separate parts. Non-identical twins are made from two separate eggs.

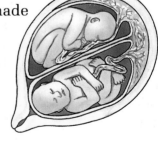

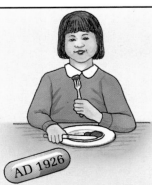

AD 1926

People suffering from anaemia (not enough iron) are cured by eating liver.

AD 1927

The 'iron lung' is used on patients whose lungs do not work on their own.

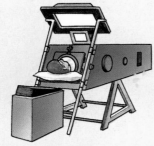

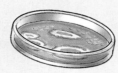

AD 1928

Alexander Fleming discovers that the bacteria penicillium destroys other bacteria. This results in the development of the world's first antiobiotic drug, pencillin.

AD 1929

Christian Eijkman of The Netherlands and Sir Frederick Hopkins of Britain win the Nobel Prize for Medicine for their work with vitamins.

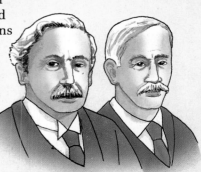

Growing up

Your body changes as you grow up. You become taller and stronger and your body changes shape. When you reach your teens you are no longer a child. You are becoming an adult.

From the time you are born you quickly grow bigger and stronger. You learn to do more and more things.

At 3 months, a baby can lift up its head and shoulders.

At 9 months, a baby can sit without help.

At 12-14 months a baby begins to walk.

At 2 years old a child is talking and beginning to play with other children.

At 3-4 years old a child can run and jump. He or she can draw pictures and get dressed without help.

Puberty

The time during which your body changes is called puberty. Girls start puberty at 10-12 years old. Boys begin later, at 12-14 years old.

A girl's breasts begin to develop and the body becomes more rounded. Body hair begins to grow.

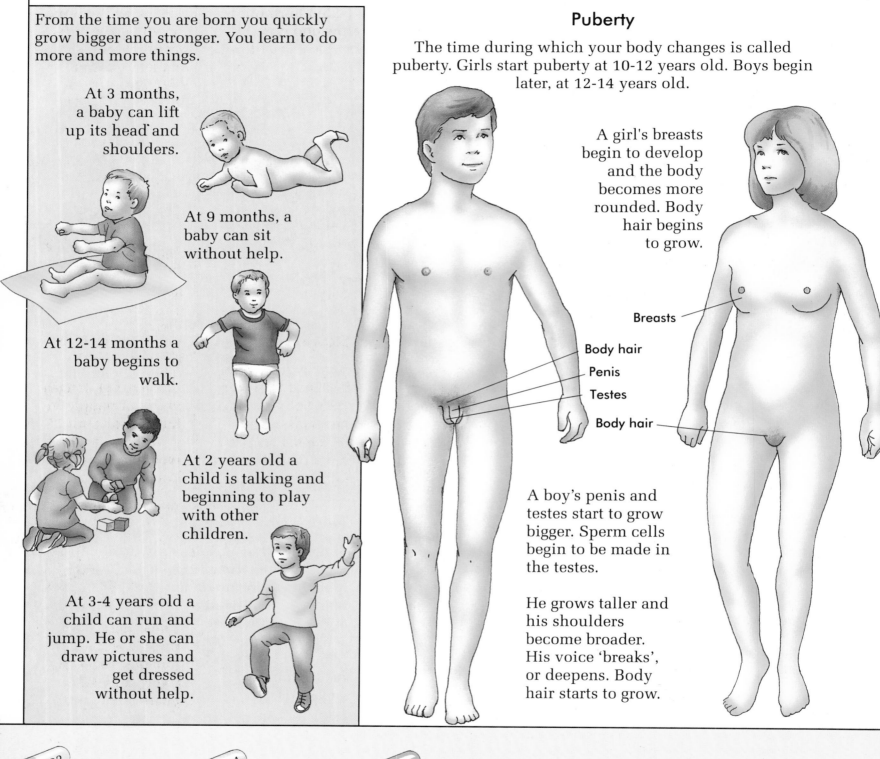

Breasts

Body hair

Penis

Testes

Body hair

A boy's penis and testes start to grow bigger. Sperm cells begin to be made in the testes.

He grows taller and his shoulders become broader. His voice 'breaks', or deepens. Body hair starts to grow.

 AD 1903

The electrocardiograph is used to measure the body's heartbeat.

AD 1904

Ivan Pavlov of Russia wins the Nobel Prize for Medicine for his study of digestion.

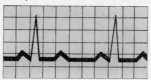

AD 1906

In New York, a carrier of typhoid germs known as 'Typhoid Mary' is found after a long hunt. She worked as a cook and passed on the illness to over 50 people.

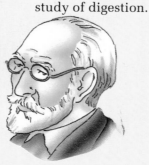

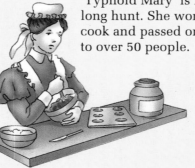

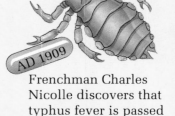 AD 1909

Frenchman Charles Nicolle discovers that typhus fever is passed on by body lice.

The most important change for girls is that they begin to menstruate (have periods). Once a month, one of the ovaries releases an egg. Unless the egg joins with a sperm (see pages 24-25) it passes out of the body together with the uterus lining.

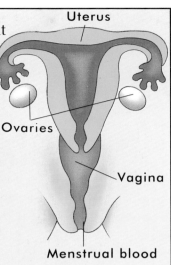

Uterus
Ovaries
Vagina
Menstrual blood

Two sets of teeth

People grow two sets of teeth in a lifetime. Your first teeth are called milk teeth. Between the ages of five and twelve, these teeth fall out and permanent teeth grow in their place.

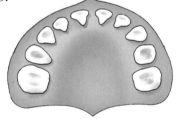

A row of 10 first, or milk, teeth.

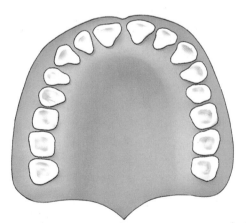

You grow more second, or permanent, teeth.

Feelings

The changes which happen to your body during puberty can make your moods go up and down very quickly. This is because the chemicals called hormones that tell your body to grow and change during puberty, also affect your emotions.

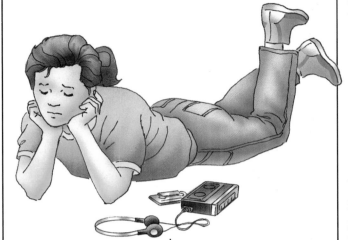

Growing older

People's bodies stop growing by about the age of 20. From then on they slowly start to age! Muscles gradually grow weaker and bones grow harder. Skin stretches and begins to wrinkle.

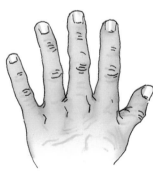

Slow down

As you grow older it takes longer for your body to make new cells. Any damage, such as a broken bone, takes longer to mend.

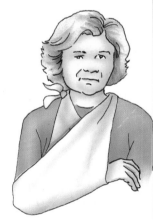

White hair

Your hair contains a special chemical called melanin, that gives it colour. As you grow older, less melanin is made. Your hair may turn grey or white.

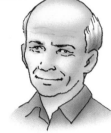

Some men go bald. When hairs die, new ones do not grow to replace them.

Lifespan

The average length of life of people in Europe is about 75 years. However, women usually live longer than men.

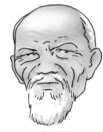

The oldest ever person was a Japanese man. He lived to be 120 years old!

AD 1911

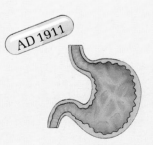

Dr William Hill invents the gastroscope, a tube that is swallowed by a patient so the doctor can look inside a patient's stomach.

AD 1915

Epidemics of tetanus break out in the trenches during World War One.

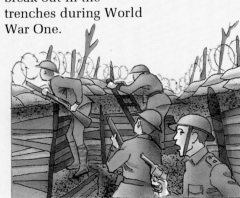

AD 1918

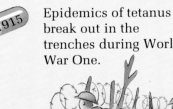

An epidemic of flu sweeps the world. In two years, 22 million people die, more than were killed throughout World War One.

AD 1921

London's first birth control clinic is opened by Dr Marie Stopes.

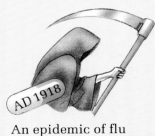

Staying healthy

To be healthy, you need to eat the right food, to exercise regularly and to rest. You also need to keep your body clean. When you are healthy, you feel good and you have lots of energy for working and playing.

Food as fuel

Food is used as fuel for your body. The nutrients it contains keep you healthy. Some foods help your body to grow and repair itself, other types are used to give you energy. To stay healthy, you need a mixture of these foods.

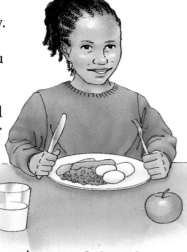

Powerful protein

Protein is found in meat, fish, eggs, cheese, milk, beans and nuts. It is used by your body to make new body tissues and to repair any damaged cells.

Careful with carbohydrates

Carbohydrates are found in potatoes, rice, bread and cakes. When you eat these foods the carbohydrate is broken down and used for energy. If you eat too many of these foods, however, the carbohydrate turns into fat!

Enough exercise

Exercise makes your body strong. It helps to protect you from illness and makes you happy and relaxed!

Vitamins and minerals

You need vitamins for your body to work properly. Vitamin C is found in fresh fruit and vegetables. It keeps your gums healthy and helps to heal wounds. Minerals, such as calcium and iron, are found in minute amounts in many foods. They keep your body working properly.

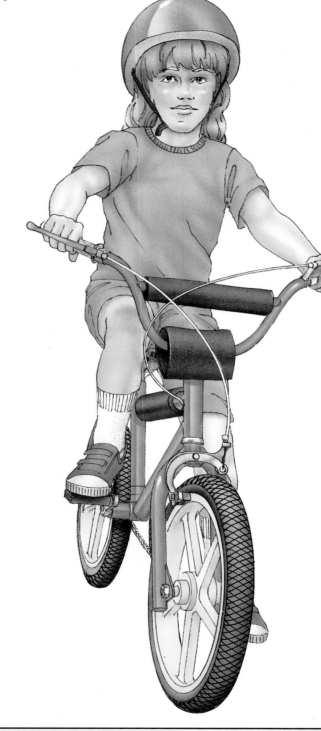

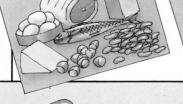

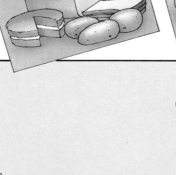

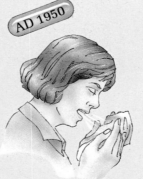

The first successful kidney transplant is performed.

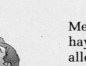

Medicines for relieving hayfever and other allergies are developed.

The structure of DNA, the chemical code that controls how life grows and reproduces, is discovered by Francis Crick and James Watson.

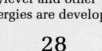

The first studies are made showing that smoking cigarettes leads to lung cancer.

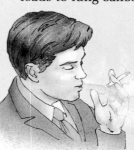

Fatty fats

Fats are found in meat, milk, butter, cheese, vegetable oils and nuts. Fats give your body energy. Fats also help to make up your cells.

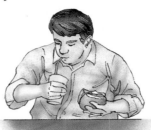

Too much fat in your body will make you put on weight! The risk of a heart attack is also higher, as fat can block up the arteries.

Water, water

You need to drink to replace the water your body loses when you sweat, breathe out and go to the toilet. All drinks contain water. Food contains water too - lettuce is 90% water!

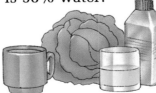

Fantastic fibre

Fibre is found in vegetables, fruit and bread. It is a carbohydrate, but one that your body cannot digest very easily. It helps to keep the muscles of your intestines working, stopping you from becoming constipated (unable to go to the toilet). This is important for good health. The longer faeces stay inside your intestines, the more water is taken back into the bloodstream, making you feel sluggish or even ill.

Clean up!

Keeping clean is an important part of staying healthy. You should have a bath or a shower every day, and always wash your hands after going to the toilet, to get rid of any germs.

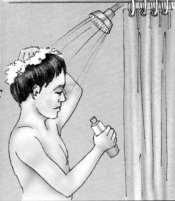

Too salty

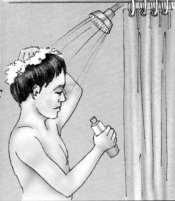

Salt helps control the amount of water in your body. It is important that you have enough of it, especially in hot weather when you sweat water and salt out of your body. However, some people believe that eating too many salty foods is not good for your health.

Time to rest

It is important to get enough rest. This is the time when damaged cells can repair themselves.

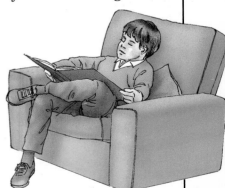

AD 1954

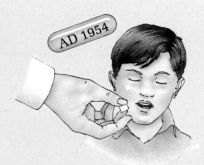

The first tests of a polio vaccine, invented by Jonas Salk of the USA, are successful. It is given to millions of children.

AD 1955

Ultrasound scanners are used to examine unborn babies in the uterus.

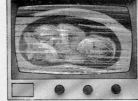

AD 1955

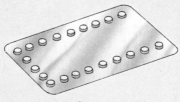

The contraceptive pill is invented.

AD 1956

A long thin tube, called an endoscope, can be used to examine the inside of the body without surgery. It is made with fibre optics and lights up so the doctor can look through it.

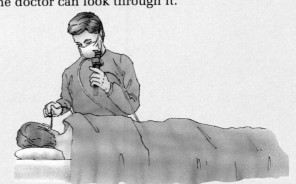

Illness

When a part of your body is not working properly you become ill. Throughout history, people have tried to discover how diseases start and how to cure them. Today, doctors are able to prevent or cure many illnesses that used to kill people in the past.

Tiny but dangerous!

Bacteria (or germs) are very tiny cells which live everywhere. They are so small that you can only see them with a strong microscope. Certain types of bacteria can cause diseases when they enter your body.

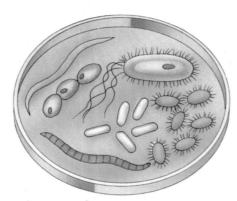

Some bacterial diseases are pneumonia, whooping cough and tonsillitis. These diseases can be treated with antibiotic medicine such as penicillin which kill bacteria.

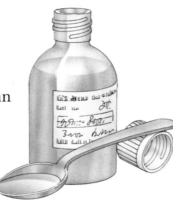

Natural defence

When you have recovered from an infectious disease, your body is now immune to it. It is unlikely that you will have the disease again.

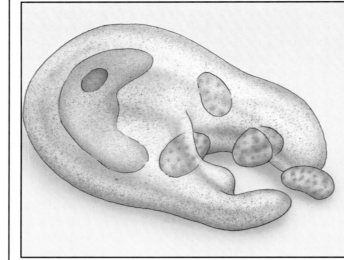

Defending cells

Your blood contains red blood cells and white blood cells. The white blood cells fight any harmful bacteria or viruses that enter your blood stream. They are part of your body's own defence system.

Deadly viruses

Viruses are even smaller than bacteria. They can only grow inside living cells, damaging them and making you ill. Some viral diseases are measles, mumps, chicken pox, the 'flu and the common cold. They are infectious diseases, easily passed from person to person.

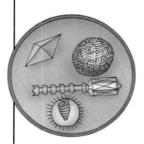

Viruses cannot be treated - it is up to our own bodies to fight them!

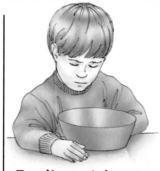

Feeling sick

There are many reasons why you are sick, or vomit. Sometimes, your body is getting rid of unwanted food, or poisons. Your stomach muscles squeeze strongly, sending the contents of your stomach upwards!

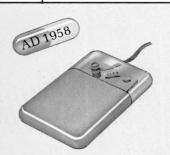

AD 1958

The first pacemaker is fitted inside a patient's chest. It keeps the heart beating at a steady pace.

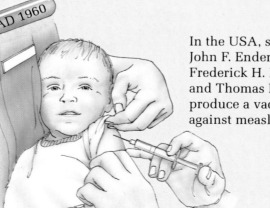

AD 1960

In the USA, scientists John F. Enders, Frederick H. Robbins and Thomas H. Weller produce a vaccine against measles.

AD 1967

The first human heart transplant is performed by South African surgeon Christiaan Barnard.

AD 1971

The first computerised brain scanners are used.

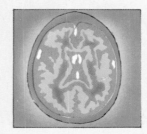

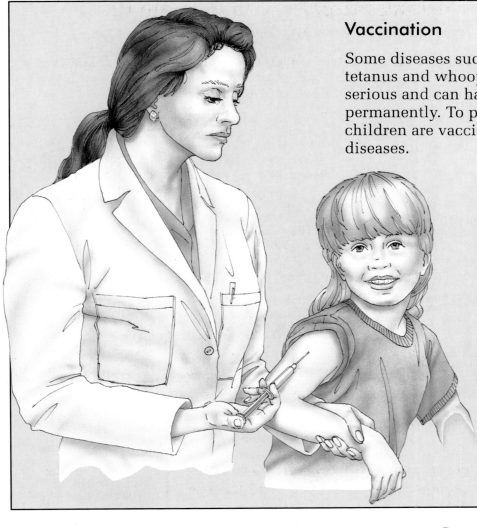

Vaccination

Some diseases such as diptheria, polio, tetanus and whooping cough, are very serious and can harm your body permanently. To protect them, most children are vaccinated against these diseases.

Vaccination is when you are injected with a weak form of a disease-causing virus or bacteria. Your body makes antibodies to fight the disease. The antibodies then stay permanently in your bloodstream.

Hot and bothered!

Sometimes, when you are ill, you feel very hot. Your body temperature goes up because you are fighting an illness. Your normal body temperature is about 37°C . This can be measured by a thermometer under your tongue or by holding a strip thermometer on the forehead.

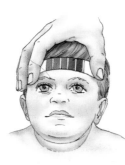

Tooth decay

Many children suffer from tooth decay. This is when plaque (a mixture of saliva, food particles and bacteria) acts with sugar to form acid. The acid attacks the tooth and eventually it may even die.

Cleaning your teeth properly at least twice a day, visiting the dentist regularly, and avoiding too many sweet drinks and sugary foods all helps to prevent tooth decay.

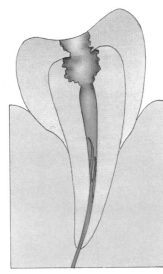

A tooth attacked by acid

Self-harm

Sometimes people cause their own illnesses. Anyone who smokes tobacco, drinks too much alcohol, or takes drugs can cause serious harm to his or her body. Smokers breathe in chemicals that can cause lung disease or cancer. Illegal drugs, such as heroin, cocaine or LSD do great harm to the body. Taking too much (an overdose) can kill. Too much alcohol damages the liver. People can often become addicted to it.

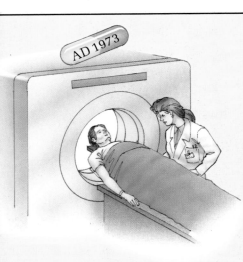

AD 1973

Body scanners take 3-D pictures of inside the human body.

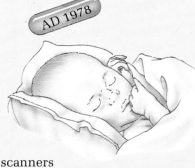

AD 1978

Louise Brown, the first baby to be conceived in a test-tube, is born.

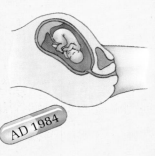

AD 1984

An operation is carried out on a baby still in the uterus.

AD 1990s

Research into genes to pinpoint the defects that cause such serious diseases as cystic fibrosis.

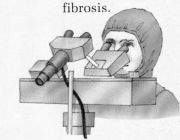

Index

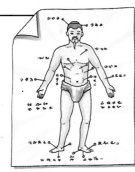

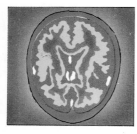
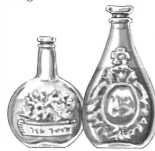
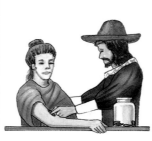
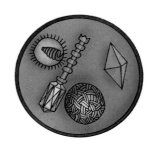
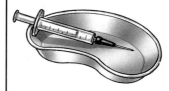
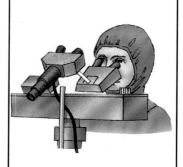